Quick and Easy Pescatarian Cookbook

Stay Healthy and fit or lose weight quickly with this beautiful mix of pescatarian recipes

Lara Dillard

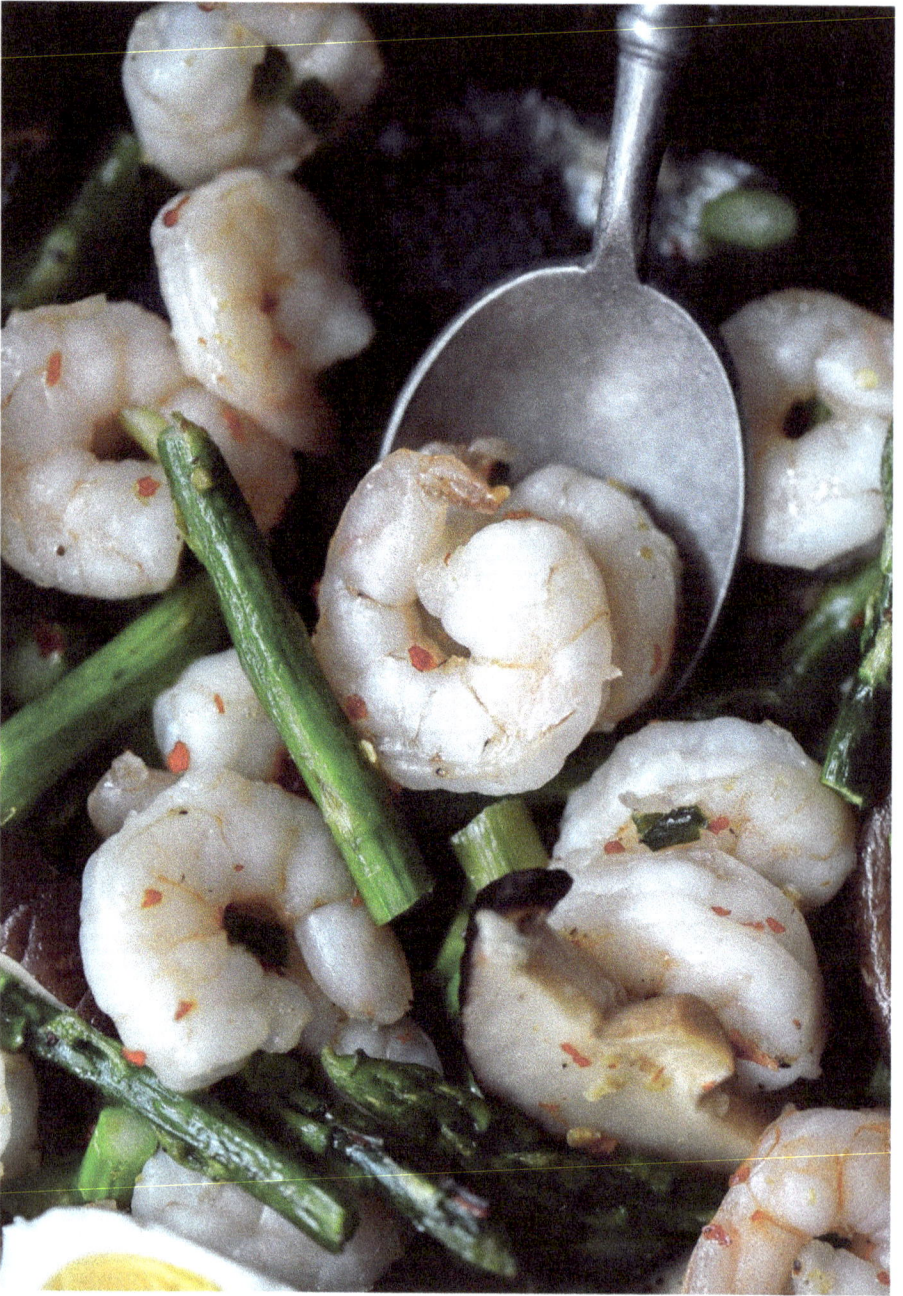

Table of Contents

Spicy Baked Shrimp

Ingredients

- 2 tsp. low-sodium soy sauce
- Pinch of cayenne pepper
- 1 lb. large shrimp, peeled and deveined
- Lemon wedges
- 1/2 cup olive oil
- 2 tablespoons Cajun seasoning
- 2 tablespoons fresh lemon juice
- 2 tablespoons chopped fresh parsley
- 1 tablespoon maple syrup

Directions

1. Preheat oven to 450 degrees F (230 degrees C).
2. Coat an 11 x 7-inch baking dish with cooking spray.
3. Mix maple syrup, olive oil, dried parsley, cayenne pepper, Cajun seasoning, lemon juice, and soy

sauce in dish

4. Add shrimp and toss to coat.

5. Bake for 8 minutes or until shrimp turn pink, stirring occasionally. Garnish with lemon wedges

6. Serve!

Maple Glazed Salmon with Wasabi

Preparation time: 40 Minutes

Ingredients

- 1 lb. salmon fillet, cut into 4 equal pieces
- 1/2 cup Mirin (Japanese sweet rice wine)
- 1 tsp. fresh ginger, peeled and minced
- 2 tablespoons soy sauce
- 1 tbsp. honey
- 2 tsp. wasabi, paste
- 1 tbsp. seasoned rice vinegar
- Salt to taste
- 2 tsp. wasabi, paste
- 1 tablespoon finely grated peeled fresh ginger
- 1/4 cup scallion, thinly sliced
- 1/2 tsp. Pepper

Directions

1. Bring vinegar, maple syrup, ginger, mirin, soy sauce, and wasabi to boil in a small saucepan, to make sauce
2. Cook, stirring occasionally, over medium-high heat until the flavors are blended and the sauce is thickened, about 5 minutes.
3. Remove from the heat and cover. Ensure it is kept warm
4. Sprinkle salmon with salt and pepper.
5. Spray a large nonstick skillet with nonstick spray and set over high heat.
6. Add salmon and cook for about 4 minutes on each side, turning once, or until the fish is browned on the outside and opaque in the center.
7. Spoon sauce over the salmon. Sprinkle with scallions and serve.

Walleye Vegetarian Delight

Servings: 4

Calories: 600

Fat: 33.4 g

Protein: 32.8 g

Carbs: 43.8 g

Ingredients and Quantity

- 4 walleye fillets
- 1/2 tbsp. lemon juice
- 1/2 cup white wine
- 1/2 tbsp. orange juice
- 1/8 cup almond butter

For the Vegetable Stuffing:

- 1/2 cup onion, chopped
- 1/4 carrots, thinly sliced
- 1/2 celery, chopped
- 1/2 green pepper, chopped
-

- 1/4 cup almond butter
- 1 cup seasoned bread crumbs
- 1 cup diced tomato
- 1/8 tsp. salt
- 1/8 tsp. pepper

Direction

1. Place the fillets on a well-greased shallow baking pan.
2. Drizzle with lemon and orange juice.
3. Cover with vegetable stuffing, wine and several slices of butter.
4. Cover with foil and bake at 350 degrees F for 20 minutes.
5. Uncover and continue to bake for 10 to 15 minutes or until fish flakes apart easily with a fork.
6. For the vegetable stuffing; sauté onion, carrots, celery and green pepper in butter until tender, about 10 minutes.
7. Add the remaining ingredients and mix well. Serve and enjoy!

Fish Stuffed Green Pepper

Servings: 4

Calories: 272

Fat: 14.5 g

Protein: 12.5 g

Carbs: 24.4 g

Ingredients and Quantity

- 2 large green peppers
- 2 tbsp. almond butter
- 2 tbsp. flour
- 1/4 tbsp. salt
- Dash pepper
- 1 cup coconut milk
- 1 cup cooked, flaked walleye, yellow perch or other fish
- 1/3 cup celery, chopped
- 1/4 cup bread crumbs

Direction

1. Cut green peppers in half, remove seeds and set aside.
2. Melt butter in a saucepan over low heat.
3. Mix in flour, salt and a dash of pepper. Add milk.
4. Cook over moderate heat, stirring constantly, until mixture thickens.
5. Remove from heat and add fish and celery.
6. Pour mixture into halved green peppers.
7. Top with bread crumbs.
8. Bake at 400 degrees F for 15 minutes. Serve and enjoy!

Oriental Fish with Sweet and Sour Vegetable

Servings: 4

Calories: 748

Fat: 31.8 g

Protein: 36 g

Carbs: 82 g

Ingredients and Quantity

- 2 lb. fish fillets, any firm fleshed fish
- 1 tbsp. lemon juice
- 1 tbsp. vegetable oil
- 2 cups julienne cut carrots
- 1/2 cup onion, thinly sliced
- 2 tbsp. water
- 2 cups sliced celery
- 1/2 cup sliced water chestnuts

- 1 can (8 1/4 oz.) pineapple chunks
- 1 1/2 tbsp. brown sugar
- 3 tbsp. cider vinegar
- 1 1/2 tbsp. soy sauce
- 1 1/2 tbsp. cornstarch

Direction

1. Place fish fillets in a skillet with enough boiling water to barely cover them. Then add lemon juice.
2. Cover and simmer for 8 to 10 minutes until fish flakes apart easily with a fork.
3. Meanwhile, heat vegetable oil in another skillet.
4. Add carrots and onions, stir fry for 5 minutes over moderately high heat.
5. Reduce to moderate heat, add water, cover and steam for 4 minutes.
6. Uncover, add celery and water chestnuts, stir fry for two minutes.

7. Add undrained pineapple.

8. Stir sugar, vinegar, soy sauce and cornstarch slowly into skillet while cooking.

9. Stir until sauce coats vegetables and pineapple.

10. Remove fish from liquid, drain well.

11. Serve topped with sweet-sour vegetable mixture. Enjoy!

Lake Erie Grill-Out

Servings: 6

Calories: 459

Fat: 27.8 g

Protein: 22.6 g

Carbs: 32.1 g

Ingredients and Quantity

- 2 lb. fish fillets (walleye, smallmouth bass or freshwater drum) 1/2 cup
- 3 tbsp. lemon juice
- 3 tbsp. liquid smoke
- 2 tbsp. Vinegar
- 1 tbsp. Salt
- 2 tbsp. Worcestershire sauce
- 1/2 tbsp. grated onion
- 1 clove garlic, finely chopped or 1 tablespoon garlic powder

- 3 drops hot pepper or Tabasco sauce (optional)

Direction

1. Cut fillets into serving size pieces.
2. Place in single layer in shallow baking dish.
3. In a separate bowl, combine remaining ingredients.
4. Pour half the mixture over fillets and marinade for 45 minutes in refrigerator, turn once.
5. Remove fish and place in a hinged wire grill.
6. Use the other half of marinade for basting.
7. Cook 4 inches from medium hot coals for 8, basting frequently.

8. Turn, baste again and cook 7 to10 minutes longer or until fish flakes apart easily with a fork

Fish Hash

Servings: 2

Calories: 529

Fat: 33.6 g

Protein: 21.7 g

Carbs: 38.3 g

Ingredients and Quantity

- 1 cup cold cooked fish fillets
- 1 cup cold boiled potatoes
- 1 large onion, grated
- 1/4 tsp. sage
- 1 egg, beaten
- 3 tbsp. almond butter
- Minced parsley, green onions or ketchup, for serving

Direction

1. Cut the sweet potatoes into small pieces and flake the fish.
2. Add onion, sage and beaten egg.
3. Melt butter in a large frying pan.
4. When hot, press the hash in and cook over medium heat until crusty brown underneath.
5. Invert on to a hot platter and sprinkle to taste with minced parsley, green onions or ketchup. Serve and enjoy!

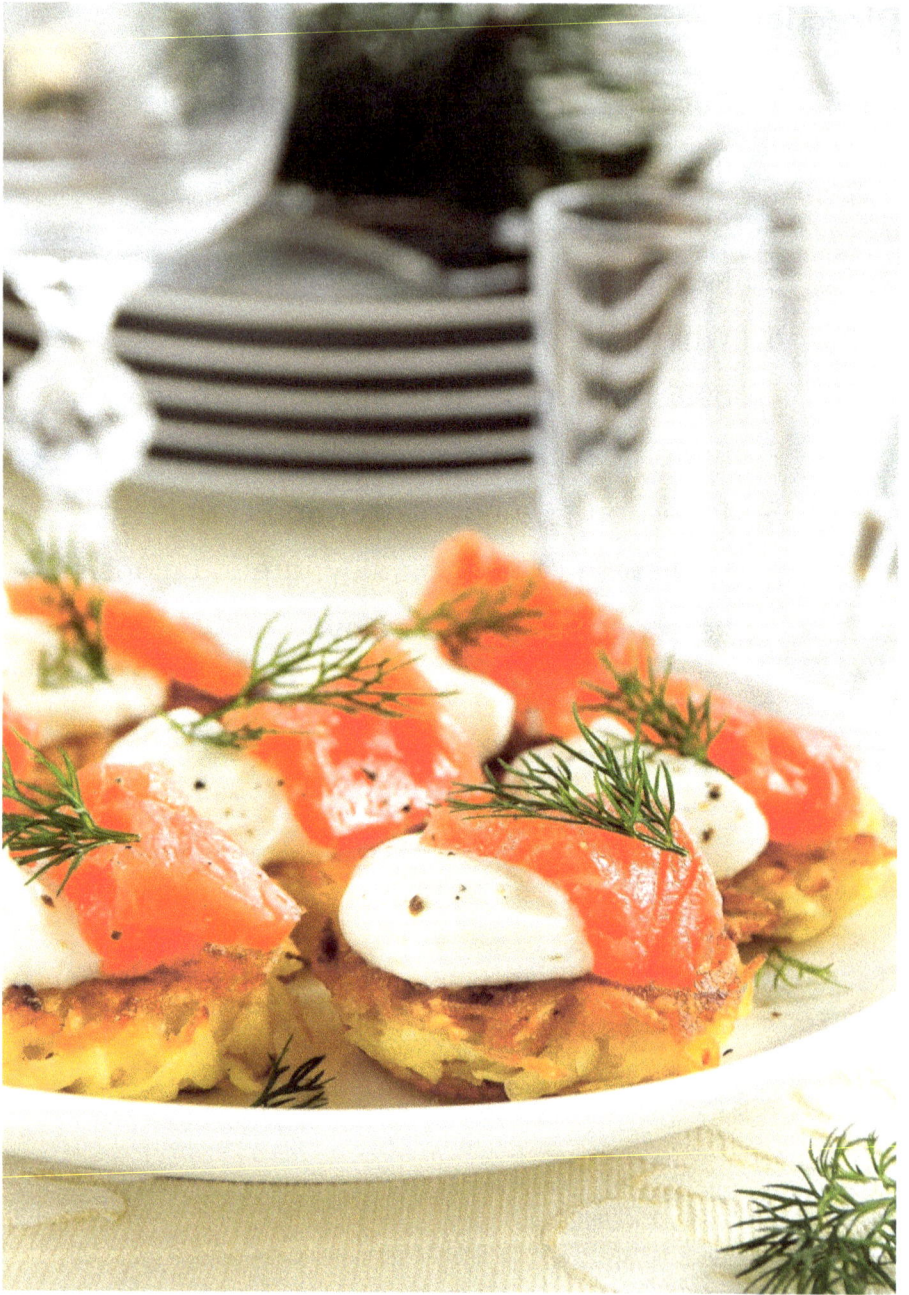

Fish Burgers

Servings: 2

Calories: 375

Fat: 22.1 g

Protein: 17.8 g

Carbs: 26 g

Ingredients and Quantity

- 1 lb. ground fish
- 1 tbsp. lemon juice
- 1/4 cup flour
- 1/2 tsp. Salt
- 1/8 tsp. pepper
- 1/2 vegetable oil
- 6 split, heated hamburger buns
- 6 lettuce leaves
- 2 tbsp. vegan mayonnaise
- 6 tomato slices

Direction

1. Sprinkle ground fish with lemon juice.
2. Mix flour, salt and pepper.
3. Cover the fish with the flour mixture.
4. Panfry in 1/4 inch hot oil until burgers are lightly browned.
5. In each bun arrange crisp lettuce, fish patty, mayonnaise and a slice of tomato. Serve and enjoy!

Baked Whole Fish with Mushrooms

Servings: 6

Calories: 686

Fat: 34 g

Protein: 73.4 g

Carbs: 17.8 g

Ingredients and Quantity

- 3 1/2 lb. whole striped bass or rainbow tout
- 1/2 cup flour
- 1/8 tsp. salt
- 1/8 tsp. pepper
- 3 tbsp. extra virgin olive oil
- 2 tbsp. almond butter
- 1 rib celery, thinly sliced
- 1 medium carrot, thinly sliced

- 1 can (8 oz.) mushrooms, thinly sliced
- 1/4 cup parsley, minced
- 2 tbsp. dry white wine
- 1/4 tsp. salt and pepper
- 1 1/3 cups spaghetti sauce with mushrooms
- ¼ cup green onions, sliced Lemon wedges, for garnishing

Direction

1. Coat fish with flour and then sprinkle with 1/8 tsp. salt and pepper.
2. Sauté in oil and butter in large skillet until brown, and then remove it.
3. Sauté celery, carrots, mushrooms, parsley, wine, 1/4 tsp. salt and pepper for 5 minutes.
4. Spread 2/3 of the celery mixture on oven-proof platter and then spoon 2/3 cup sauce over it.
5. Stuff fish with remaining celery mixture and then arrange on platter.
6. Spoon remaining sauce on fish.

7. Bake at 425 degrees F until fish is tender, about 20 minutes.

8. Sprinkle with green onions and then garnish with lemon. Serve and enjoy

Citrus Marinated Fish Fillets

Servings: 2

Calories: 371

Fat: 15.7 g

Protein: 42.7 g

Carbs: 18.7 g

Ingredients and Quantity

- 1 pound fresh or frozen fish fillets
- 2/3 cup lime juice
- 2 tbsp. vegetable oil
- 4 tsp. maple syrup
- 2/3 cup water
- 1 tsp. dried dill weed
- 1/2 tsp. salt

Direction

1. Thaw fish, if frozen.

2. Separate fillets or cut into 4 serving-sized portions.
3. Put fish in a shallow pan.
4. For marinade, mix lime juice, vegetable oil, maple syrup, water, dill weed and salt.
5. Divide marinade into 2 equal portions, reserve and store one portion in refrigerator.
6. Pour the other portion of marinade over the fish.
7. Cover and refrigerate for 3 hours or overnight, turning fish occasionally.
8. Remove fish from the pan, disposing of used marinade.
9. Place fish on slightly greased rack of a broiler pan.
10. Broil fish 4 inches from heat until fish flakes easily when tested with fork, allow 5 minutes for each 1/2-inch thickness.
11. Baste fish often with reserved portion of marinade during broiling. Serve and enjoy!

Southern Bass Chowder

Servings: 4

Calories: 427

Fat: 18.5 g

Protein: 53.6 g

Carbs: 10 g

Ingredients and Quantity

- 1/4 cup almond butter
- 1 tbsp. flour
- 1/2 cup scallions, chopped
- 1 garlic clove, minced
- 1/4 cup green pepper, chopped
- 1/2 cup celery, chopped
- 1/2 cup zucchini, chopped
- 1 can (16 oz.) tomatoes
- 1/2 cup dry sherry
- 1 tbsp. lemon juice
- 3 tbsp. tabasco sauce
- 1/8 tsp. salt and pepper

- 1/2 tbsp. thyme
- 2 lb. bass fillets

Direction

1. Melt the butter in skillet.
2. Blend in flour and stir over heat for 2 minutes.
3. Add scallions, garlic, green pepper, celery and zucchini, and then cook until vegetables are soft.
4. Chop tomatoes into small pieces and add to skillet.
5. Combine all other ingredients except fish, and mix well.
6. Simmer uncovered for 1 1/2 hours, adding a little water if necessary, stirring occasionally.
7. Place fish fillets on top of sauce.
8. Cover and increase heat.
9. Cook for 10 minutes or until fish flakes apart easily with a fork.
10. Serve over rice or grits. Enjoy!

Seasoned Fish

Servings: 9

Calories: 366

Fat: 24.2 g

Protein: 14 g

Carbs: 24.4 g

- **Ingredients and Quantity**
- 1/2 package (6 oz. package) oyster crackers, crushed
- 1/2 tsp. lemon pepper
- 1/2 tsp. seasoned salt
- 1/2 cup vegetable oil
- 1 tsp. dill weed
- envelope (1 oz.) Hidden Valley salad dressing
- 9 fish fillets

Direction

1. Mix together crackers, lemon pepper, salt, oil, dill weed and salad dressing.
2. Preheat oven to 375 degrees F.
3. Pour 1/2 cup oil onto a cookie sheet with sides, until bottom is covered.
4. Put cookie sheet in oven while coating fish.
5. Coat fish fillets with cracker mixture.
6. Put fillets on cookie sheet when oil is hot and return to oven.
7. Turn fillets several times until golden brown, or fry 6 1/2 minutes on each side. Serve and enjoy!

Lemon Fish Roll Ups

Servings: 8

Calories: 377

Fat: 23.7 g

Protein: 18.7 g

Carbs: 23.9 g

Ingredients and Quantity

- 1/3 cup almond butter
- 2 tsp. salt
- 1/3 cup lemon juice
- 1 1/3 cups cooked white rice
- 1 cup sharp cheddar cheese, shredded
- package (10 oz.) frozen broccoli, thawed, chopped
- 8 fish fillets
- Paprika, for topping

Direction

1. In small saucepan, melt butter.
2. Add salt, pepper and lemon juice. Set aside.
3. In medium bowl, combine rice, cheese, broccoli and 1/4 cup of the lemon mixture.
4. Place 1/8th of the rice mixture on top of each of the 8 fish fillets and roll the fillets up.
5. Place seam-side down in 11x7-inch baking dish.
6. Top with remaining sauce, then sprinkle with paprika.
7. Bake at 375 degrees F for 25 minutes or until fish flakes with fork. Serve and enjoy!

Fish in Creole Sauce

Servings: 6

Calories: 981

Fat: 25.2 g

Protein: 113.8 g

Carbs: 67.1 g

Ingredients and Quantity

- 2 tbsp. almond butter
- 1/4 cup onion, chopped
- 1 garlic clove, minced
- 6 green olives, minced
- 2 cups stewed tomatoes
- 1/2 green pepper, chopped
- 1/2 bay leaf
- 3 beef bouillon cubes
- 1/8 tsp. Thyme
- 2 tsp. parsley, chopped

- 1 tsp. Sugar
- 1/3 tsp. Salt
- Cayenne pepper to taste
- 1/4 cup white wine
- 1/4 cup mushrooms, sliced
- 5 Northern pike fillets, boned and cut in 2 inches chunks
- 25 frozen medium shrimp
- 6 cups cooked rice

Direction

1. Melt the butter and sauté onion, garlic and olives about 2 minutes.
2. Add and cook the rest of the ingredients, except the fillets and shrimp, until sauce is thickened, about 50 minutes.
3. Add fillet chunks and 20 to 25 frozen shrimp to the sauce and cook for 15 minutes or until fish is well cooked.
4. Serve over hot rice. Enjoy!

Easy Fish 'N' Chips

Servings: 4

Calories: 598

Fat: 36.7 g

Protein: 18.9 g

Carbs: 45.3 g

Ingredients and Quantity

- 1/2 cup almond butter
- 2 potatoes, peeled and cut in 1/4 inch slices
- 3/4 cup Ritz crackers, crushed
- 2 tbsp. parsley
- 1 tsp. paprika
- 3/4 tsp. salt
- 1/2 tsp. garlic powder
- 1 lb. frozen fish fillets, thawed

Direction

1. Melt butter 9 by 13 inch pan.
2. Add potato slices and stir to blend.
3. Cover with foil and bake at 350 degrees F for 20 to 25 minutes.
4. Combine crackers, parsley, paprika, salt and garlic powder.
5. Spoon potatoes to one side of baking dish.
6. Dip fillets into melted butter that potatoes were in; then roll in crumb mixture.
7. Place fillets in same baking dish with potatoes.
8. Sprinkle with remaining crumb mixture.
9. Return to oven and continue baking, uncovered for 20 to 30 minutes.
   Serve and enjoy!

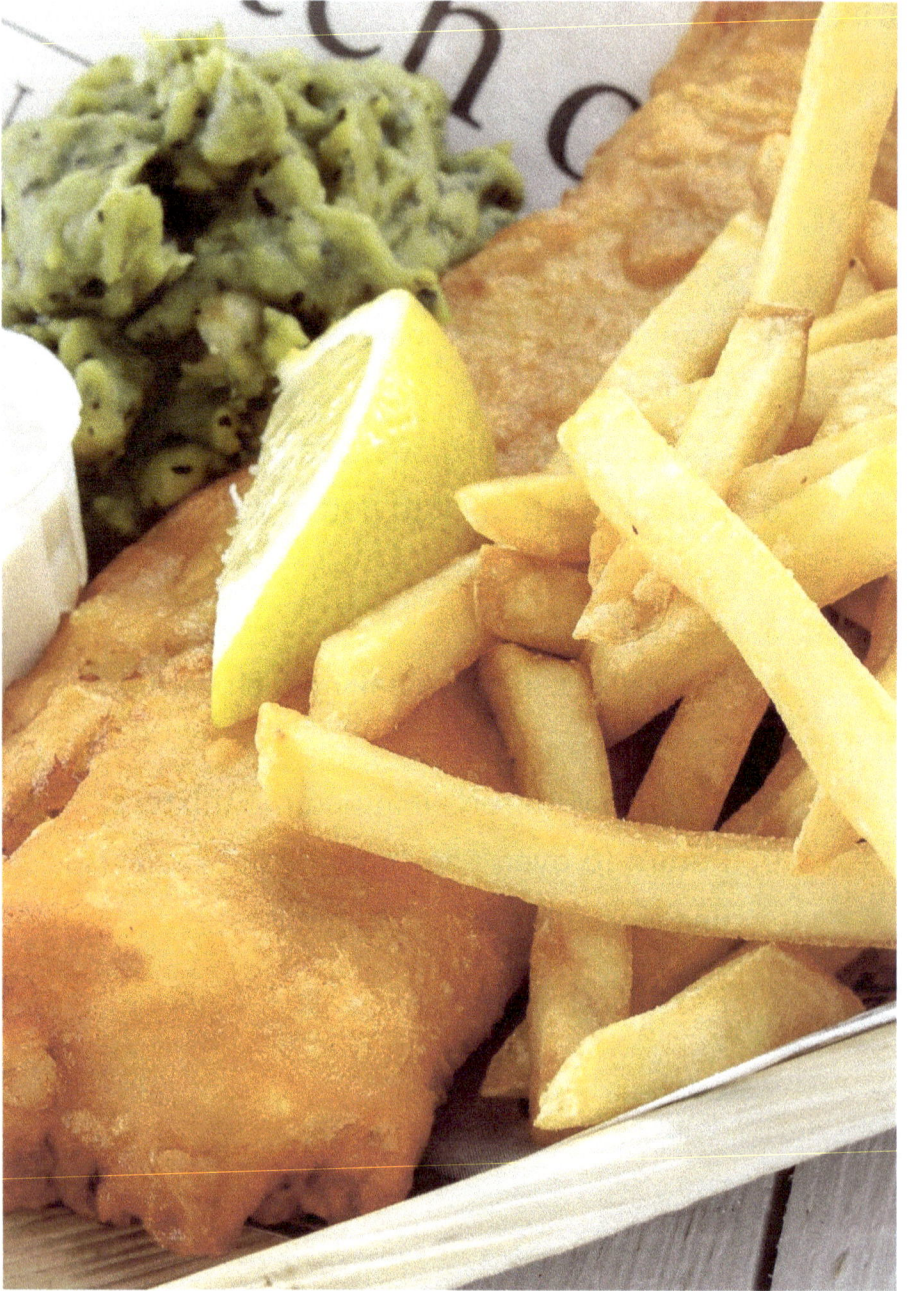

Easy Baked Fillets

Servings: 4

Calories: 277

Fat: 16.2 g

Protein: 14.8 g

Carbs: 19.7 g

Ingredients and Quantity

- 4 fish fillets
- 1 cup shrimp, cooked and deveined
- 4 tbsp. mayonnaise
- 4 slices lemon
- Aluminum foil

Direction

1. Cut 4 large rectangles of aluminum foil.
2. Put one fillet on each rectangle.

3. Add 1/4 cup shrimp on top of each fillet and 1 tbsp. mayonnaise on top of that.
4. Wrap foil around fish tightly and bake at 375 degrees F for 10
5. minutes or until fish flakes easily with fork.
6. Serve with a slice of lemon. Enjoy!

Broiled Fish with Dijon Sauce

Servings: 3

Calories: 532

Fat: 33.5 g

Protein: 24.9 g

Carbs: 35.8 g

Ingredients and Quantity

- 3 tbsp. vegan cheese, freshly grated
- 2 tbsp. Dijon mustard
- 1/2 cup mayonnaise
- 1/8 tsp. black pepper
- 1 lb. firm fish fillets

Direction

1. In a bowl, mix the cheese, mustard, mayonnaise and pepper.

2. Spread cheese mixture on the fillets.

3. Broil the fillets for 4 to 7 minutes, depending on the size and thickness of the fish, or just until the fish flakes with a fork. Serve and enjoy!

Baked Fish Fillets

Servings: 4

Calories: 383

Fat: 20.1 g

Protein: 18.1 g

Carbs: 34.2 g

Ingredients and Quantity

- 1 lb. fish fillets
- 2 tbsp. lemon juice
- 2 tbsp. almond butter, melted
- 1/4 tsp. dill weed
- 1/2 tsp. Salt
- 1/4 tsp. Pepper
- 2 cups Total cereal, crushed

Direction

1. Grease baking pan.
2. If the fillets are large, cut into serving sizes.
3. Mix lemon juice and butter; reserve.
4. Mix dill weed, salt and pepper.
5. Dip each fillet in butter mixture; sprinkle with salt mixture and coat with cereal.
6. Bake, uncovered, at 350 degrees F for 20 to 30 minutes or until fish flakes easily. Serve and enjoy!

Fillet Almondine

Servings: 4

Calories: 453

Fat: 29.9 g

Protein: 18.5 g

Carbs: 28 g

Ingredients and Quantity

- 1/3 cup almonds, sliced or silvered
- 1/4 cup almond butter
- 1 pound lean fish fillets
- 1/2 tbsp. salt
- 1 tbsp. dry white wine or lemon juice

Direction

1. Place almonds and the butter in a 9-inch pie plate.
2. Microwave on high for 3 to 5 minutes until almonds are golden, stirring twice.
3. Remove almonds with a slotted spoon and set aside.
4. Add fillets to butter, turning to coat.
5. Arrange fillets in dish with thicker portions towards the outside of dish.
6. Cover with wax paper.
7. Microwave on high 4 to 6 minutes, until fish begins to flake when fork is inserted in thickest part.
8. Sprinkle with salt, wine or lemon juice and reserved almonds. Serve and enjoy!

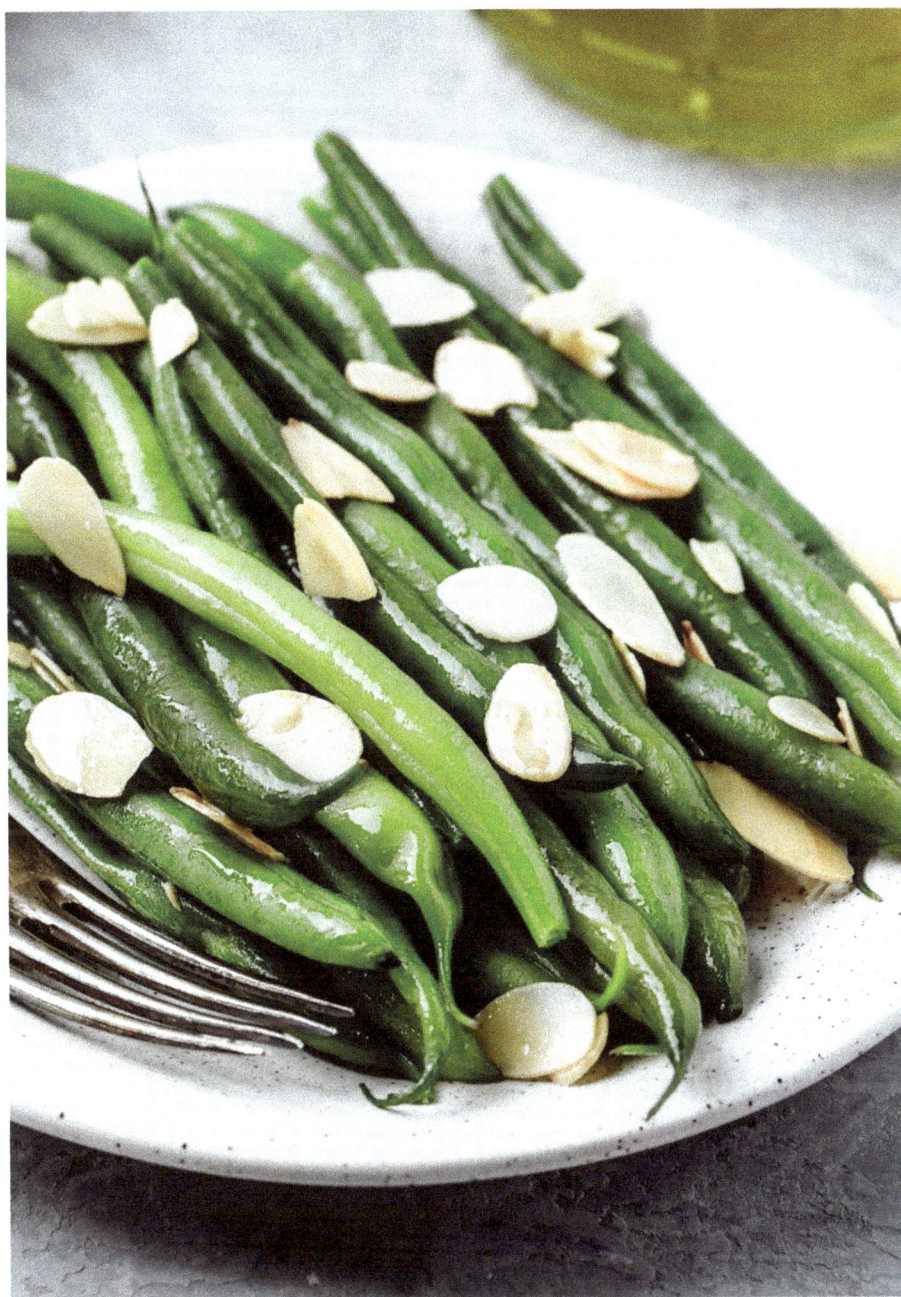

Fish Fillets in Foil

Servings: 4

Calories: 477

Fat: 14.5 g

Protein: 20.3 g

Carbs: 66 g

Ingredients and Quantity

- 4 fillets of fish
- 4 pieces aluminum foil
- 1 cup salsa
- 4 cups hot cooked white rice
- Lime wedges, for garnish
- Nonstick cooking spray

Direction

1. Using a nonstick spray, spray 4 pieces of foil.
2. Place a fish fillet on each foil.

3. Top with 1/4 cup salsa.

4. Fold foil, crimping edges tightly to seal.

5. Cook on a hot barbecue grill for about 10 minutes.

6. Remove from grill and open foil packet carefully to avoid the hot steam.

7. Serve each fillet with the sauce on rice and garnish with lime wedges. Enjoy!

Chili Green Beans

Servings: 4

Total Time: 25 Minutes

Calories: 161

Fat: 3.7 g

Protein: 1.5 g

Carbs: 6.9 g

Fiber: 2.5 g

Ingredients and Quantity

- 1 1/2 cup green beans
- 1 red onion, chopped
- 1 red chili pepper, minced
- 1 tsp. hot paprika
- 2 tomatoes, chopped
- 1 tsp. tomato paste
- 1 tsp. black pepper

- 1 tsp. salt
- 1 cup water
- 1 tbsp. olive oil

Direction

1. In the instant pot, mix the green beans with the onion, pepper and the other ingredients and toss.
2. Close and seal the lid. Set Manual mode (High pressure) and cook green beans for 8 minutes.
3. Then allow natural pressure release for 5 minutes.
4. Open the lid and mix up the green beans carefully. Serve and enjoy!

Zucchini Lasagna

Servings: 2

Total Time: 31 Minutes

Calories: 308

Fat: 13.2 g

Protein: 10.4 g

Carbs: 10.8 g

Fiber: 5.5 g

Ingredients and Quantity

- 3 oz. almonds, crushed
- 1/4 tsp. salt
- 1/2 tsp. black pepper
- 1 tbsp. water
- 1 tsp. olive oil
- 1/2 tsp. lemon juice
- 6 oz. tomatoes, diced and canned
- 3 oz. kale

- 1 zucchini
- 1 tsp. dried oregano
- 1 tsp. Italian seasoning
- 1 onion, grated

Direction

1. In the food processor blend together almonds, salt, water, and olive oil.
2. When the mixture is smooth, transfer it in the mixing bowl.
3. After this, blend lemon juice with diced tomatoes, dried oregano, Italian seasoning, and grated onion.
4. Cut the zucchini lengthwise. The "lasagna" noodles are prepared.
5. Then place little bit tomato mixture in the bottom of the instant pot.
6. Place one zucchini slice and spread it with cashew mixture.
7. Repeat the same steps till you use all the ingredients.

8. Close and seal the lid. Set High-pressure mode and cook the meal for 9 minutes.

9. Then allow natural pressure release for 9 minutes.

10.   10. Open the lid and chill the lasagna till it reaches room temperature. Serve and enjoy!

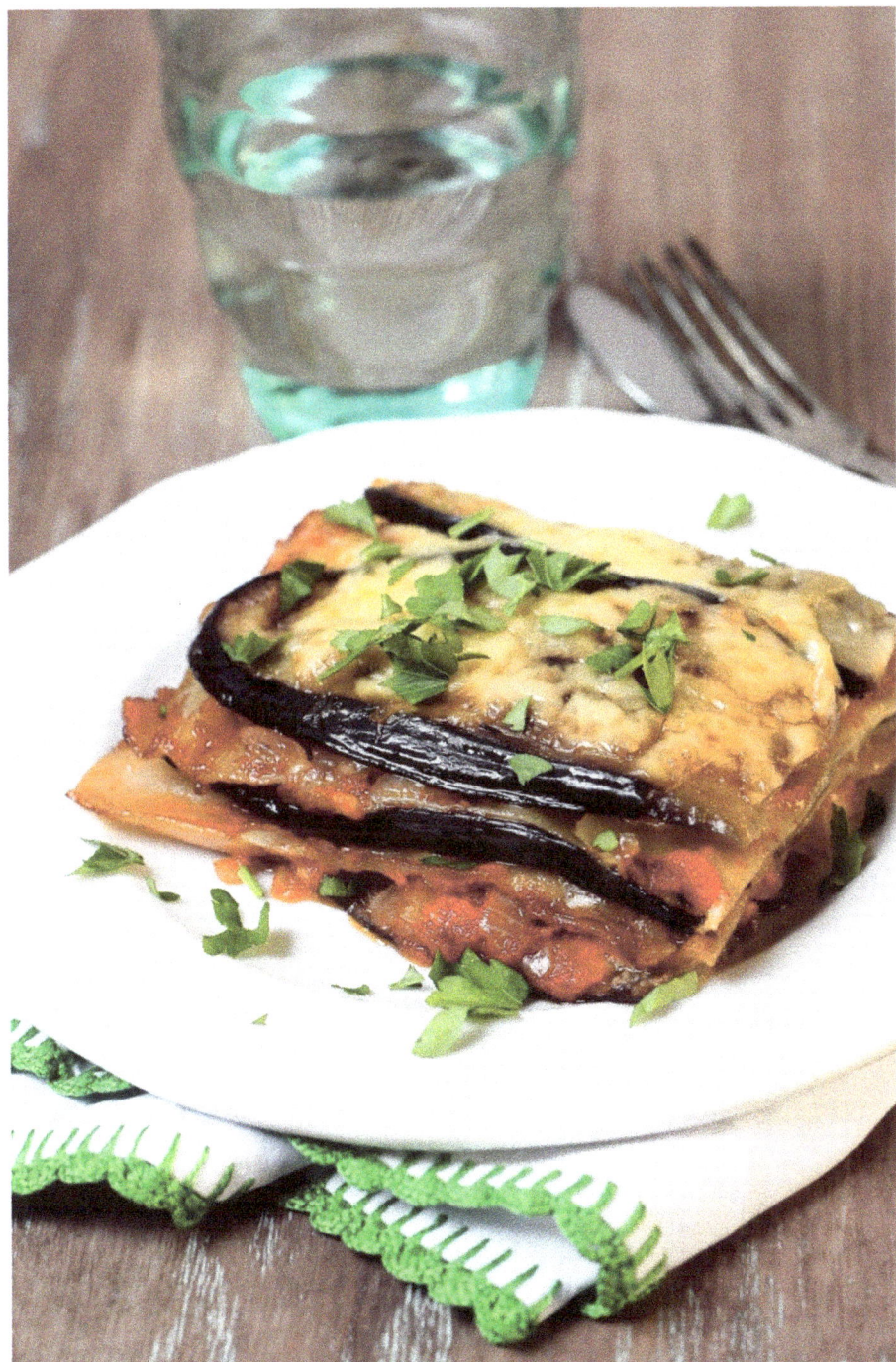

Ginger Tofu

Servings: 2

Total Time: 20 Minutes

Calories: 261

Fat: 16.9 g

Protein: 22.6 g

Carbs: 10.4 g

Fiber: 2.5 g

Ingredients and Quantity

- 1 pound firm tofu, roughly cubed
- 1 tsp. minced garlic
- 11/2 tsp. minced ginger
- 6 tbsp. soy sauce
- 1 tsp. avocado oil
- 1 tbsp. balsamic vinegar
- 1/2 tsp. brown sugar

- 1/2 tsp. red chili pepper
- 1/4 cup water

Direction

1. In the instant pot, mix the tofu with the garlic, ginger and the other ingredients. Toss gently and close the lid.
2. Set Manual mode (high pressure) and cook a meal for 5 minutes.
3. Make a quick pressure release.
4. Transfer the cooked meal into the serving bowls and top with the gravy. Serve and enjoy!

Tofu and Sauce

Servings: 4

Total Time: 13 Minutes

Calories: 245

Fat: 19.8 g

Protein: 12.8 g

Carbs: 8.4 g

Fiber: 2.9 g

Ingredients and Quantity

- 10 oz. firm tofu, cubed
- 1/4 cup vegetable stock
- 1 tsp. turmeric powder
- 1 tsp. basil, dried
- 1/2 tsp. Salt
- 1 tsp. ground black pepper
- 1 tbsp. avocado oil

- 1/2 tsp. corn flour
- 4 tbsp. coconut butter
- 5 tbsp. almond yogurt
- 1/2 tsp. curry powder
- 1 tbsp. soy sauce
- 1/4 cup peanuts, chopped
- 1/2 tsp. dried rosemary

Direction

1. Sprinkle tofu with salt and place in the instant pot. Add the stock and close the lid.
2. Cook the tofu on High pressure mode for 1 minute.
3. Then use quick pressure release.
4. Add the rest of the ingredients and toss gently.
5. Close and seal the lid. Cook the meal for 2 minutes on Manual mode.
6. Then use quick pressure release.
7. Transfer the tofu into the serving plates and top with gravy. Serve and enjoy!

Lemon Soybeans

Servings: 10

Total Time: 36 Hours

Calories: 125

Fat: 5.6 g

Protein: 10.2 g

Carbs: 8.4 g

Fiber: 2.6 g

Ingredients and Quantity

- 1 1/2 cup soybeans
- 1 tsp. turmeric powder
- 6 cups water
- 1 tbsp. lemon juice
- 1 tsp. tempeh starter
- 1 cup water, for cooking

Direction

1. Place soybeans, turmeric and 5 cups water in the instant pot. Close and seal the lid.
2. Set High-pressure mode and cook soybeans for 45 minutes.
3. Then allow natural pressure release for 30 minutes.
4. Transfer the cooked soybeans in the bowl and sprinkle with lemon juice and tempeh starter.
5. Mix up the soybeans and transfer into the freezer bags. Seal them.
6. Pour the rest of the water in the instant pot.
7. Add sealed freezer bags with soybeans.
8. Close the lid and set "Yogurt" mode. Cook tempeh for 15 hours.
9. When the time is over, the tempeh should get the white color.
10. Remove the tempeh from the instant pot and let it rest for hours. Slice it into the servings. Enjoy!

Keto Seafood Chowder

Servings: 4

Total Time: 40 Minutes

Ingredients and Quantity

- 4 tbsp. almond butter
- 2 garlic cloves, minced
- 1 1/2 cups (5 oz.) celery stalks, sliced
- 1 cup clam juice
- 1 1/2 coconut cream
- 2 tsp. dried sage or dried thyme
- 1/2 lemon, juice and zest
- 4 oz. vegan cheese
- 1 lb. salmon or boneless fillets, cut into 1 inch pieces
- 2 cups (2 oz.) baby spinach
- 8 oz. shrimp peeled and deveined
- Salt and ground black pepper
- 1/2 tbsp. red chili peppers
- Fresh sage, optional, for garnishing

Direction

1. Melt almond butter in a large pot over medium heat.
2. Add garlic and celery. Cook for about 5 minutes, stirring occasionally. Add clam juice, coconut cream, vegan cheese, sage, lemon juice and lemon zest. Let it simmer for about 10 minutes without lid.
3. Add the fish and shrimp. Simmer for 3 minutes or until fish is just cooked. Add the baby spinach and stir and until wilted.
4. Season with salt and pepper, to taste.
5. Garnish with fresh red chili and fresh sage before serving for extra flavor and splash of color. Enjoy!

20 Minutes Fish Stew

Servings: 4

Total Time: 23 Minutes

Ingredients and Quantity:

- 2 tbsp. olive oil
- 1 small white onion
- 2 cloves garlic, minced
- 1 1/2 lb. wild cod
- 15 oz. can diced tomato
- 1/2 cup coconut milk
- 1/4 cup coconut cream, optional
- 2 tbsp. tomato paste
- 1 whole red, green and yellow bell pepper, sliced in rounds
- 1 pinch sea salt and ground black pepper
- 1/2 tsp. red pepper flakes
- 1 tbsp. fresh cilantro

Direction

1. Heat oil in a large skillet or cast iron. Add onion and garlic, cook until fragrant, about 3 minutes.

2. Now add diced tomatoes and stir. Add coconut milk, sour cream (optional) and tomato paste. Stir the sauce and allow to cook for about 3 minutes.

3. Add the sliced pepper and cod chunks. Then season with salt, pepper and red pepper flakes.

4. Cover and allow the fish to simmer for about 10 to 12 minutes. When the fish has cooked for about 7 to 8 minutes, carefully turn the cod so that the other side will be properly cooked in the broth.

5. When done, garnish with fresh cilantro. Serve and enjoy!

Blackened Tilapia Tacos

Servings: 4

Total Time: 23 Minutes

Calories: 266

Fat: 18.9 g

Protein: 14 g

Carbs: 3.5 g

Fiber: 3 g

Ingredients and Quantity

For the Blackened Tilapia:

- 1/2 pound tilapia
- 1 tsp. chili powder
- 1 tsp. paprika
- Salt and pepper, to taste

For the Cabbage Slaw:

- 1/2 cup red cabbage
- 1 tbsp. olive oil
- 1 tbsp. lime juice
- 1 tsp. apple cider vinegar

For the Tortillas:

- 1/2 cup flaxseed meal
- 1 tbsp. psyllium husk powder
- 1/2 cup plus 1 tbsp. water
- 2 tbsp. olive oil
- 4 tbsp. guacamole
- Spices of your choice

Direction

1. Make a half batch of flax seed tortillas.
2. Thinly chop about 1/2 cup red cabbage.
3. Use 1 tablespoon olive oil, juice of 1 lime (about 1 tablespoon) and 1 teaspoon apple cider vinegar to dress the cabbage. Mix well and set aside.
4. Use chili powder, paprika, salt and pepper to season both sides of the tilapia.
5. Add 1 tbsp. olive oil in a sauce pan and heat it up in medium heat.
6. Add the fish and cook each side for about 3 minutes. Make sure the outside is a bit blackened, but not burnt
7. Remove the fish from the pan and set aside for some time.
8. Assemble tacos by placing fish, red cabbage, guacamole and sour cream (1 tablespoon per taco). Squeeze fresh lime juice on top. Then add a bit of cilantro. Serve and enjoy!

Low Carb Flaxseed Tortillas

Servings: 4

Total Time: 30 Minutes

Calories: 184.4

Fat: 11.8 g

Protein: 5 g

Carbs: 2.2 g

Fiber: 2.4 g

Ingredients and Quantity

- 1 cup golden flaxseed meal
- 2 tbsp. phyllium husk powder
- 2 tsp. olive oil
- 1/4 tsp. xanthan gum
- 1/2 tsp. curry powder
- 1 cup plus 2 tbsp. filtered water

Per tortilla: 1 tsp. olive oil, for frying and 1/2 tsp. coconut flour for rolling.

Direction

1. In a mixing bowl, add 1 cup golden flaxseed meal, 2 tbsp. psyllium husk powder, 1/4 tsp. xanthan Gum and 1/2 tsp. curry powder or spices of your choice.
2. Mix all of the dry ingredients together well.
3. Now add 2 tsp. olive oil and 1 cup plus 2 tbsp. filtered water to the mixture. Mix well until a solid ball is formed out of the mixture.
4. Leave this ball uncovered on the countertop so that all liquid will be absorbed by the flax meal.
5. Next, measure out portions of tortillas and get a silpat ready. If using a tortilla press, measure out 5 portions. If you are rolling by hand, measure 3 to 4 portions out.
6. For each portion, press it against the silpat with your hands.
7. Sprinkle about 1/2 tsp. coconut flour over the tortilla and rolling pin. Roll out the

dough as flat as you can without tearing it.

8. Using a large round object (I used the lid of a pan), cut out your tortilla and separate it from the excess dough. You can use the excess dough to roll out more tortillas.

9. You will have a perfectly round tortilla. Repeat this process for each tortilla.

10. Place a pan over medium-high heat and add 1 tsp. olive oil.

11. Add the tortilla and fry until brown once the oil is hot.

12. You can add fillings of your choice. Serve and enjoy!

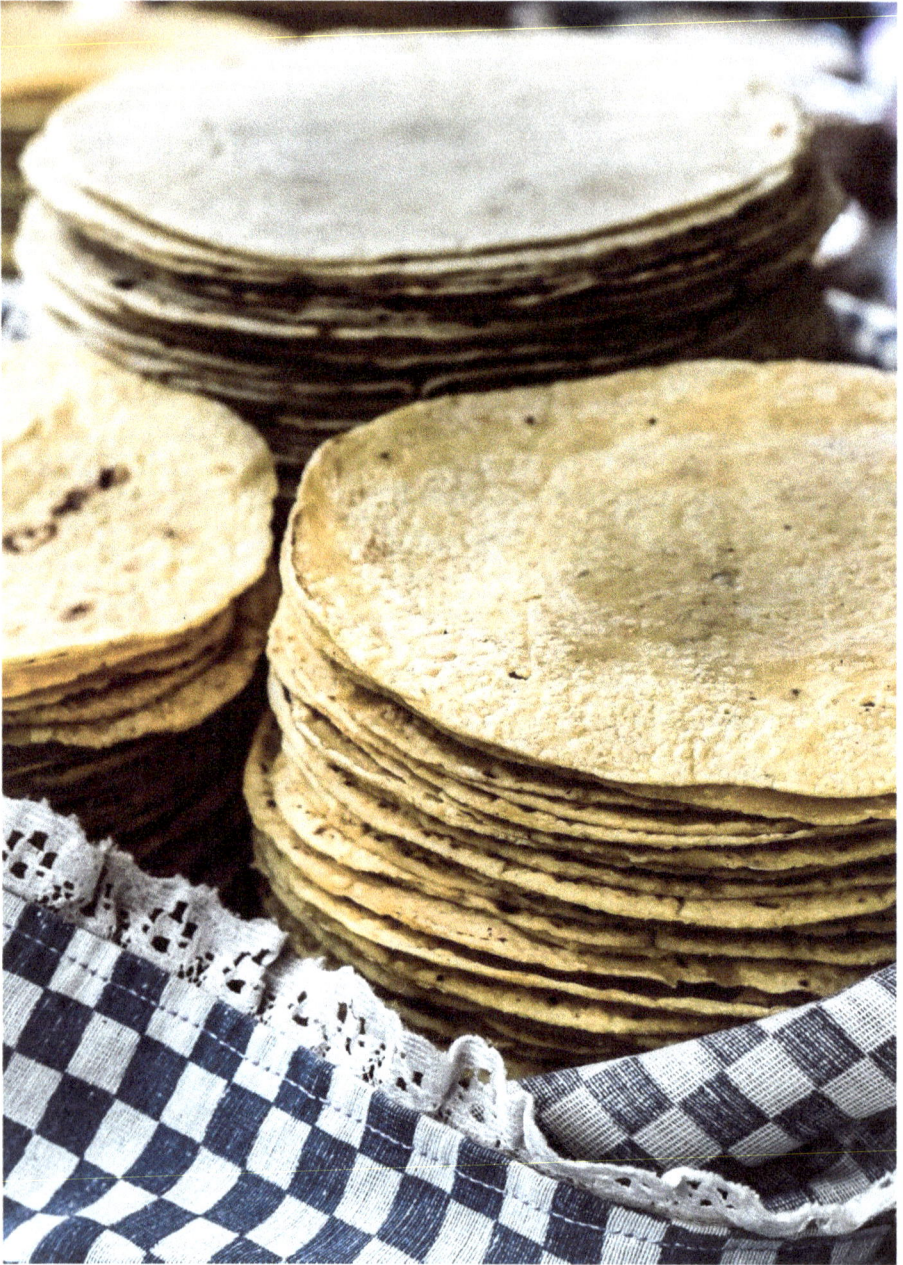

Low Carb Keto Fish and Chips

Servings: 2

Total Time: 45 Minutes + 2 Hours Marinating Time

Calories: 242

Fat: 13 g

Protein: 26 g

Carbs: 1 g

Fiber: 1 g

Ingredients and Quantity

For the Keto Fish Tacos:

- 250 g firm white-flesh fish, preferably cod 1/3 cup coconut cream
- 2 tsp. apple cider vinegar
- 4 cloves garlic, ran through a press
- Kosher salt, to taste
- 1/2 cup whey protein isolate

- 1 tsp. baking powder
- 1/4 tsp. garlic powder
- 1/4 to 1/2 tsp. kosher salt, to taste
- 3 tbsp. apple sauce
- 2 tsp. apple cider vinegar
- Coconut oil, or any other healthy cooking oil of your choice

Optional Serving Suggestions:

1 batch jicama fries, 8 tortillas

1 batch vegan keto mayonnaise

Lemon

Vinegar

Direction

1. Mix the coconut cream, vinegar and garlic. Season to taste with salt.
2. Cut the fish across the grain of the flesh into stripes roundly, 2 inches wide and add them to the cream marinade.
3. Cover and refrigerate for 2 hours.

4. Optionally you can make a batch of keto jicama fries.

5. Add enough oil to a skillet or frying pan to make it about 1/2 inch deep. Use a narrower pan to save a lot of oil. Then heat up the oil over medium-low heat while coating the fish.

6. In a shallow dish, mix the whey protein, baking powder, garlic powder and salt.

7. In a second plate, mix the apple sauce and the vinegar.

8. Dip the fish in the apple sauce mix and then in the whey protein mix. Make sure these mixtures coat the fish properly.

9. Now place the coated fish in the hot oil and blast the top immediately.

10. Fry both sides until deep golden. Then transfer to a paper-lined plate for some minutes.

11. Serve immediately, together with the jicama fries, enough lemon, vegan keto mayo and a drizzle of vinegar. Enjoy!

Low Carb Tuna Rolls

Servings: 3

Total Time: 30 Minutes

Ingredients and Quantity

- 1 medium sized cucumber
- 1 can or pouch of tuna
- 1 tbsp. vegan mayo
- 2 tsp. sriracha
- 2 tsp. garlic powder
- Salt and pepper, to taste
- Avocado, sliced and cut to match the width of cucumber strips

For the Sauce:

- 2 tbsp. vegan mayo
- 2 tsp. Sriracha

Direction

1. Use a vegetable peeler to slice the cucumber lengthwise in order to get thin strips.
2. Drain the tuna if necessary and mix with the vegan mayo, sriracha, garlic powder, salt and pepper. Ensure that the mixture is a bit moist, but not too wet.
3. Now place the cucumber strips on prep surface and neatly spread tuna mixture tightly along leaving about 1 inch at the end of the strip.
4. Next, place avocado pieces at end of cucumber strip on top of tuna and roll tightly.
5. For the sauce, mix the vegan mayo and sriracha. Then drizzle over cucumber rolls. Serve and enjoy!

Lemon Dill Tuna Cakes

Servings: 8

Total Time: 20 Minutes

Calories: 215

Fat: 14.2 g

Protein: 22.2 g

Carbs: 1.7 g

Fiber: 0.7 g

Ingredients and Quantity

- 4 (5 oz.) cans tuna, drained
- 1/3 cup almond flour
- 3 medium green onions, chopped, white and light green parts only
- 2 tbsp. chopped fresh dill
- 1 tbsp. lemon zest
- 3/4 tsp. Salt
- 1/2 tsp. Pepper

- 1/4 cup vegan mayo
- 3 tbsp. apple sauce
- 1 tbsp. freshly squeezed lemon juice
- 2 tbsp. avocado oil

Direction

1. Mix together all the ingredients all other ingredients in a large bowl, except the avocado oil. Mix until well combined.
2. Form 8 patties from the mixture, about 3/4 inch thick.
3. Heat 1 tbsp. avocado oil in a large skillet over medium heat until shimmering. Then add half of the tuna patties. Cook for about 3 to 4 minutes, or until golden brown on the bottom
4. Flip the patties over carefully and cook the other side for another 3 to 4 minutes.
5. Transfer to a paper towel-lined plate. Repeat for the remaining oil and patties.
6. Now top the patties with vegan mayo, lemon and capers (optional). Serve and enjoy!

Tuna Stuffed Avocados

Servings: 4

Total Time: 15 Minutes

Calories: 478

Fat: 39 g

Protein: 23.3 g

Carbs: 12.8 g

Fiber: 9.6 g

Ingredients and Quantity

- 4 medium size avocados
- 2 (5 oz.) cans tuna
- 1/4 cup vegan mayo
- 1 celery stalk, diced
- 2 tbsp. red onion, diced
- 1/2 tbsp. chopped parsley, chives and other herbs of your choice

- 1/2 tbsp. Dijon mustard
- Salt and pepper, to taste

Direction

1. In a mixing bowl, add the tuna, mayonnaise, diced celery, diced red onion, herbs, Dijon mustard, salt and pepper. Stir together until well combined.
2. Slice the avocados in half and remove the seed.
3. Add a few spoonsful of tuna salad onto each avocado half. Serve and enjoy!

Crab Stuffed Avocado with Lime

Servings: 2

Total Time: 10 Minutes

Calories: 434

Fat: 36 g

Protein: 11 g

Carbs: 12 g

Fiber: 10 g

Ingredients and Quantity

- 1 ripe California avocado, halved and pitted
- 1/4 cup avocado   oil mayonnaise
- 3 tbsp. plus 1 tsp. fresh lime juice, divided
- 2 tbsp. diced onion
- 2 tbsp. chopped fresh cilantro
- 1/2 tsp. ground cumin
- 1/4 tsp. fine sea salt

- Ground pepper, to taste
- 1 (6 oz.) can crab meat (I used lump crab meat)
- Lime wedges, for serving
- Dash sriracha, optional

Direction

1. Combine the mayonnaise, 3 tbsp. lime juice, onions, cilantro, cumin, salt and pepper in a medium bowl. Gently fold in the crabmeat. Adjust seasoning to taste.
2. Use the remaining lime juice to brush the avocado, to avoid browning.
3. Place avocado halves, cut side up, on plates. Add the crab salad into each avocado half.
4. Serve with lime wedges and dash of sriracha, if desired. Enjoy!

Keto Fried Shrimp

Servings: 8

Total Time: 30 Minutes

Calories: 475

Fat: 37 g

Protein: 30.5 g

Carbs: 4.8 g

Fiber: 2.3 g

Ingredients and Quantity

For the Shrimp:

- 350 g peeled raw shrimp (12.4 oz.)
- 1/2 tsp. Dijon mustard
- 1 1/2 tsp. paprika
- 1/2 tsp. thyme
- 1 tsp. garlic powder
- 1/2 tsp. cayenne pepper

- 1 tsp. dried oregano
- 3/4 cup whey protein powder
- 5 tbsp. apple sauce
- 1 tbsp. coconut cream
- 1/2 tsp. hot sauce, or to taste
- 1 tsp. flaked sea salt
- 1/4 tsp. cracked black pepper
- 2 cups avocado or coconut oil, for frying

For the Slaw:

- 2 cups shredded white cabbage
- 1 cup shredded red cabbage
- 1 medium celery, sliced
- 1 medium spring onion, sliced
- 2 tbsp. vegan mayo
- 1 tsp. lemon juice
- Pinch sea salt

Direction

1. In a bowl, mix the dry ingredients: paprika, thyme, garlic powder, cayenne pepper, oregano, pinch of salt and whey protein powder.
2. In another bowl, mix the wet ingredients: apple sauce, coconut cream, hot sauce, Dijon mustard and a pinch of salt.
3. Dip the shrimp in the wet mixed ingredients and then in the dry ingredients. Shake off the excess ingredients. Do this in small batches of 5 shrimps at a time to avoid clumping.
4. Add the avocado or coconut oil to a deep pan (about 7.5 inches) that will allow the shrimp to be completely submerged.
5. Heat up the oil and then fry the shrimp on a medium-low heat for about 1 to 2 minutes or until golden and cooked through. Do the frying in batches of 5 shrimps at a time for even frying and no clumping.

6. Use a slotted spoon to drain the shrimp from the oil. Use a paper towel to absorb excess oil while frying the other batches.

7. For the slaw, simply mix all the ingredients together in a bowl.

8. Serve the fried shrimp with the slaw. Optionally, you can serve with a vegan mayo. Enjoy!

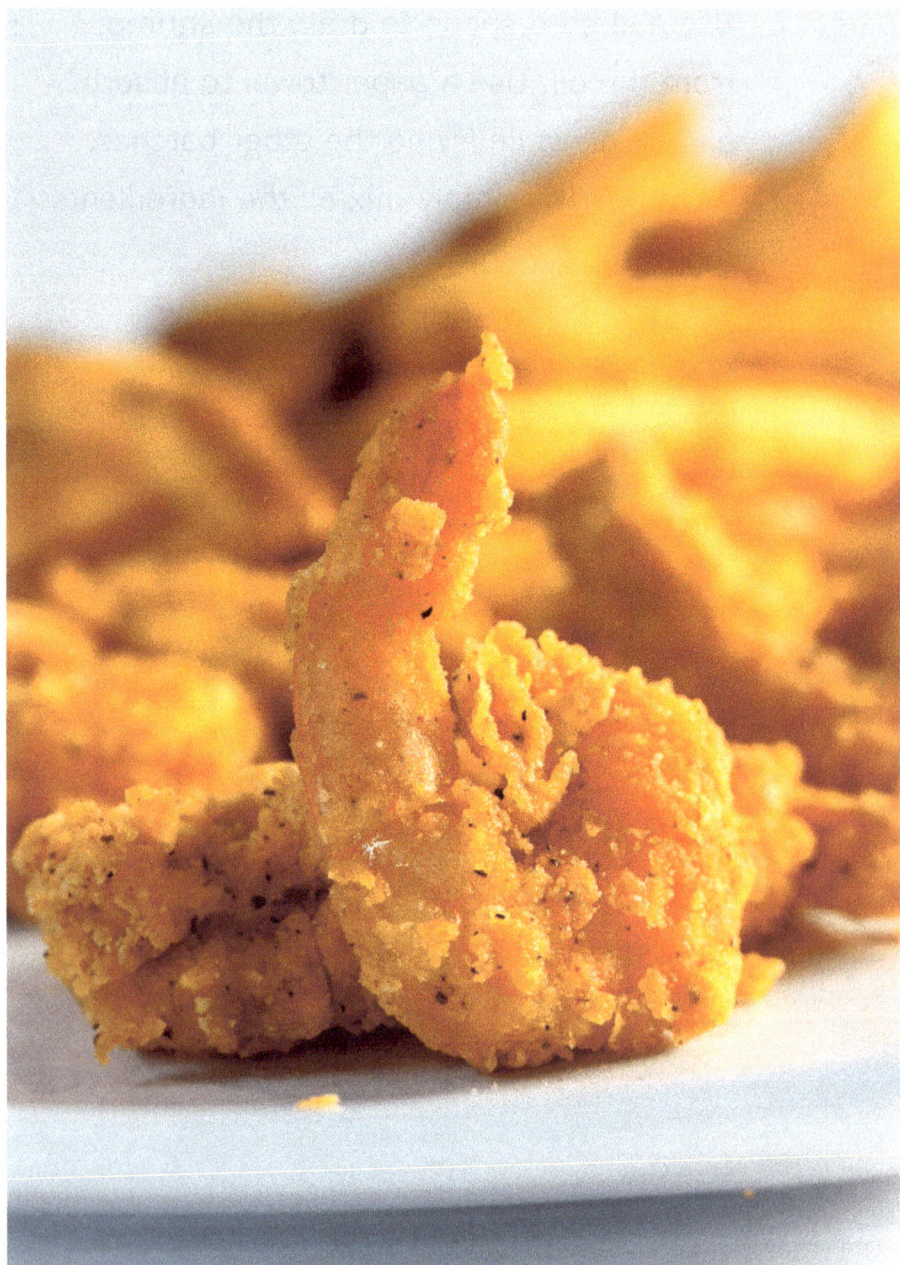

Crispy Cod with Keto Cheese Sauce and Broccoli

Servings: 4

Total Time: 20 Minutes

Calories: 433

Fat: 29.3 g

Protein: 34.9 g

Carbs: 6.4 g

Fiber: 2.3 g

Ingredients and Quantity

For the Cheese Sauce:

- 2 tbsp. coconut cream
- 1 tbsp. almond butter
- 2 tbsp. vegan cheese
- Pinch sea salt, optional

- 1 tbsp. water, or more if you need to thin it down

For the Cod and Broccoli:

- 1 (250 g) small bunch broccoli
- 2 skin-on cod loins (300 g)
- Sea salt and pepper, to taste
- 1 tbsp. avocado oil

Direction

1. To make the cheese sauce, place the coconut cream and almond butter into a small sauce pan and gently heat up. Add the vegan cheese.
2. Stir until melted and then bring to a simmer. Once bubbles start forming, remove the heat source.
3. Mix until smooth and creamy. For a thicker sauce, you can cook for extra 3 to 5 minutes while stirring. You can add a splash of water or coconut cream.

4. Pat the cod loins dry with a paper towel. Season both sides with salt and pepper.

5. Pour the avocado oil in a skillet or a non-stick pan and heat up over medium-high heat.

6. Add the cod loins, skin side down. Cook for 3 to 5 minutes, depending on the thickness of the fish, or until the skin is crisped on and the sides are opaque. Flip the fish and cook for another 1 to 2 minutes. When done, set aside and keep warm.

7. Cut the ends off the broccoli and cut in half. Then place the broccoli florets in a double boiler or a pot filled with boiling water. Cook for 4 to 5 minutes, or until the broccoli becomes crisp-tender.

8. Serve the broccoli with the crispy cod and cheese sauce immediately. Sprinkle with more pepper to taste. Enjoy!

9. You can serve immediately or store for up to a day. But you need to reheat gently before eating the next day.

Tuscan Butter Salmon

Servings: 4

Total Time: 45 Minutes

Ingredients and Quantity

- 2 tbsp. extra virgin olive oil
- 4 (6 oz.) salmon fillets, patted dry with paper towels
- 3 cloves garlic, minced
- 1 1/2 cups halved cherry tomatoes
- 2 cups baby spinach
- 1/2 cup coconut cream
- 1/4 cup vegan cheese
- 1/4 cup chopped herbs (basil and parsley), plus more for garnishing
- Kosher salt, to taste
- Freshly ground black pepper
- Lemon wedges, for serving (optional)

Direction

1. Heat the oil in a large skillet over medium-high heat. Season the salmon all over with salt and pepper.
2. Immediately the oil starts shimmering, add the salmon, skin side up and cook for about 6 minutes or until deep golden. Flip over and cook 2 more minutes. Then transfer to a plate.
3. Reduce the heat to medium and then add the almond butter. Wait for the butter to melt and then stir in the garlic. Cook for 1 minute or until fragrant.
4. Add cherry tomatoes and then season with salt and pepper. Cook until the tomatoes begin to burst.
5. Now add spinach and cook until they begin to wilt.
6. Stir in the heavy cream, vegan cheese and hers. Then bring the mixture to a simmer.

7. Reduce the heat to low and simmer for about 3 minutes or until sauce is slightly reduced.

8. Put back the salmon in a skillet and spoon over sauce. Simmer for about 3 minutes or until salmon is cooked through.

9. Use the herbs to garnish it and squeeze lemon on top before you serve. Enjoy!

Lemon Garlic Shrimp

Servings: 4

Total Time: 15 Minutes

Ingredients and Quantity

- 2 tbsp. almond butter, divided
- 1 tbsp. extra-virgin olive oil
- 1 lb. medium shrimp, peeled and deveined
- 1 lemon, thinly sliced, plus juice from 1 lemon
- 3 cloves garlic, minced
- 1 tsp. crushed red pepper flakes
- Kosher salt
- 2 tbsp. dry white wine, or water
- Freshly chopped parsley, for garnishing

Direction

1. Melt 1 tablespoon each of almond butter and olive oil in a large skillet over medium heat.
2. Add the shrimp, crushed red pepper flakes, lemon slices, garlic and then season with salt.
3. Cook for about 3 minutes per side or until shrimp turns pink and opaque, stirring occasionally.
4. Remove the skillet containing the shrimp from the heat source and then stir in the remaining almond butter, lemon juice and white wine.
5. Season with salt and garnish with parsley before serving. Enjoy!

Keto Baked Salmon

Servings: 4

Total Time: 30 Minutes

Calories: 303

Fat: 19 g

Protein: 30 g

Carbs: 3 g

Fiber: 2 g

Ingredients and Quantity

- 1 tsp. avocado oil
- 2 tbsp. soy sauce
- 2 tbsp. rice vinegar
- 4 tsp. sesame oil
- 4 (4 to 5 oz.) salmon fillets
- 1/2 tsp. sea salt
- 1/2 tsp. black pepper
- 1/4 cup sesame seeds

- 2 tsp. fresh thyme

Direction

1. Preheat your oven to 400 F.
2. Use a paper towel to pat the salmon dry and then season it with salt and pepper.
3. Use avocado oil to lightly grease a baking dish and then place the salmon fillets in it.
4. Whisk together the soy sauce, rice vinegar and sesame oil in a small bowl.
5. Then pour the mixture over the salmon and bake for about 15 minutes, or until the salmon is fully cooked.
6. Now sprinkle the sesame seeds before serving. You can pair it with cauliflower. Serve and enjoy!

Garlic Shrimp Zoodles

Servings: 2

Total Time: 15 Minutes

Calories: 276

Fat: 10 g

Protein: 38 g

Carbs: 9 g

Fiber: 2 g

Ingredients and Quantity

- 2 medium zucchini
- 3/4 pounds medium shrimp, peeled and deveined
- 1 tbsp. olive oil
- Juice and zest of 1 lemon
- 3 to 4 cloves garlic, minced
- Salt and pepper, to taste

- Fresh parsley, chopped
- Red pepper flakes, optional

Direction

1. Use a spiralizer to spiralize the zucchini on the medium setting. Set aside.
2. In a skillet over medium heat, add the olive oil lemon juice and zest.
3. Once the pan has heat up a bit, add the shrimp and cook for 1 minute per side.
4. Add the garlic and red pepper flakes. Cook for extra 1 minute, stirring continuously.
5. Add the zucchini noodles and toss (with tongs) continuously for about 2 to 3 minutes until they are slightly cooked and warmed up.
6. Season with salt and pepper. Then sprinkle the chopped parsley on top. Serve immediately. Enjoy!

Keto Crab Cakes (Gluten-Free)

Servings: 8

Total Time: 30 Minutes

Calories: 106

Fat: 7 g

Protein: 9 g

Carbs: 12 g

Fiber: 0.4 g

Ingredients and Quantity

- 1 lb. lump crab meat
- 1/2 cup onion, finely chopped
- 3 tbsp. blanched almond flour, or golden flaxseed, for nut-free diet
- 1/4 cup apple sauce
- 2 tbsp. Worcestershire sauce
- 1 tsp. mustard

- 1 tbsp. dried parsley
- 1 tbsp. old bay seasoning
- 2 tbsp. olive oil, divided

Direction

1. In a skillet, heat 2 tbsp. olive oil over medium heat. Then sauté the chopped onion for about 10 minutes, or until translucent and lightly browned.
2. Meanwhile, mix all the other ingredients except the crab meat and the remaining olive oil, until well combined. Then add the sautéed onions. Finally, fold in crab meat very gently. Avoid breaking up the lumps of crab meat.
3. Form 8 patties and then place them on a lined baking sheet or cutting board. You can refrigerate for like 30 minutes so that the crab cakes will stay together when frying.
4. In a skillet over medium heat, fry the crab cakes in two batches. Use about 2 tbsp. olive

oil for each batch and cook for about 3 to 5 minutes per side, until browned. Serve and enjoy!

Low Carb Tuna Salad

Servings: 8

Total Time: 10 Minutes

Calories: 167

Ingredients and Quantity

- 2 (12 oz.) cans tuna, solid white Albacore in water
- 3 to 4 celery stalks, diced (about 1 1/2 cups)
- 1/3 cup shallot, small dice (1 medium shallot can serve)
- 1 1/4 cups avocado oil mayo
- 1 tbsp. celery seed
- 2 tbsp. fresh lemon juice
- 1 tsp. salt

Direction

1. Drain the tuna and add to a large bowl.
2. In a medium bowl, add all remaining ingredients and mix well.
3. Adjust the seasonings to your taste. Serve cold. Enjoy!

Cannellini Beans with Eggplant

Servings: 4

Ingredients and Quantity

- 2 medium sized eggplants, peeled and diced
- 1 can cannellini beans, drained
- 1 cup canned tomatoes, drained and diced
- 1 red bell pepper, chopped
- 1 onion, chopped
- 4 garlic cloves, chopped
- 1 bunch parsley, chopped, for serving
- 3 tbsp. extra virgin olive oil
- 1/2 tsp. paprika
- 1 green chili, chopped
- 1 tbsp. dried mint
- Salt and black pepper, to taste
- 1/2 cup finely cut fresh parsley

Direction

1. Gently sauté onion, garlic, eggplants in

olive oil on medium-high heat for 6 to 7
minutes.
2. Add in paprika and chili pepper and
cook for 1 to 2 minutes, stirring.
3. Add the rest of the ingredients.
4. Cover and simmer on low-high heat for 30
minutes.
5. Sprinkle with parsley. Serve and enjoy!

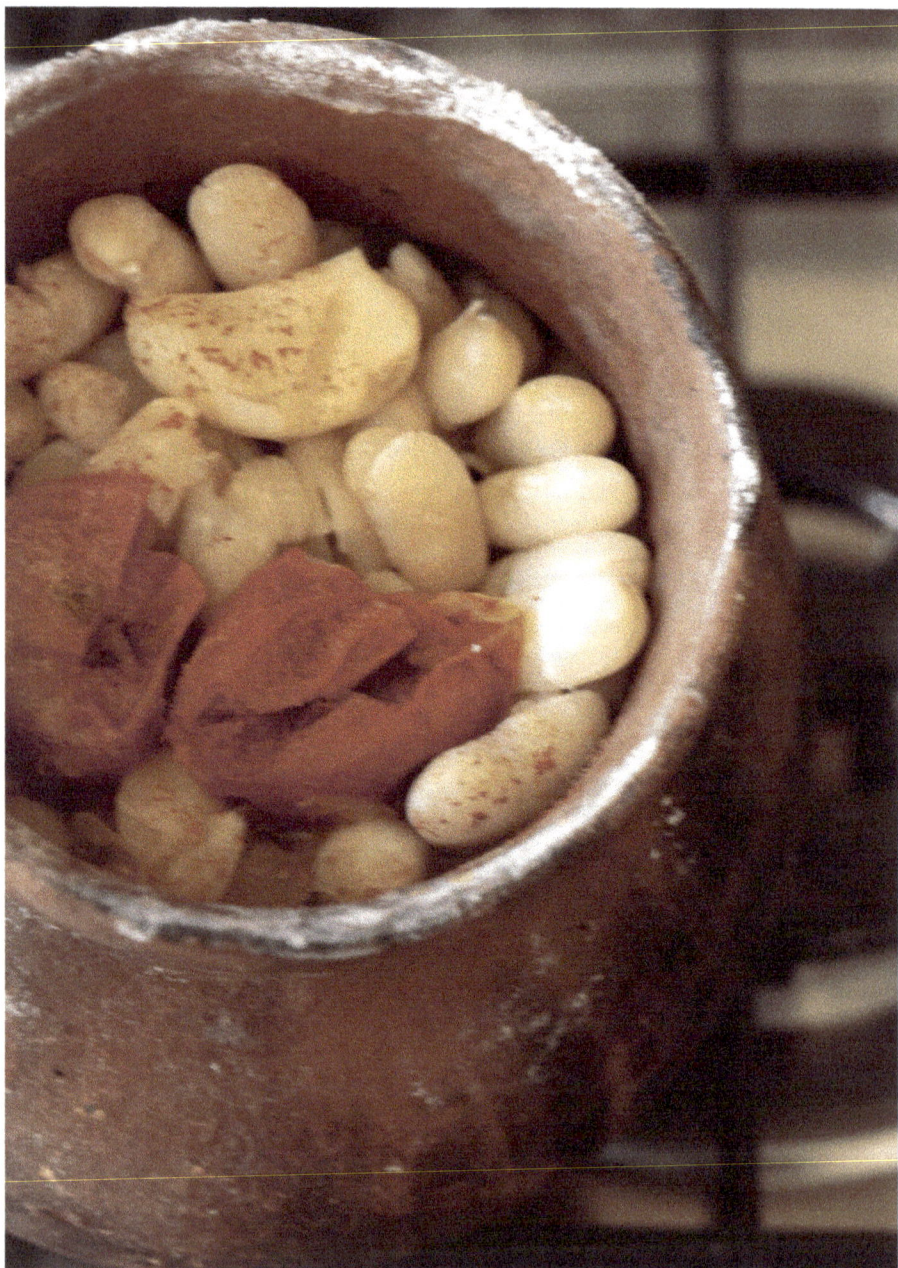

www.ingramcontent.com/pod-product-compliance
Lightning Source LLC
Chambersburg PA
CBHW050753030426
42336CB00012B/1790